UNLOCK YOUR ULTIMATE METABOLISM

ONCE AND FOR ALL

LEONIDAS PETRIDIS

CONTENTS

 This book contains only the harsh and unfiltered truth. If you want someone to sugarcoat it, this is definitely not the right place for you. I am not going to lie to you: boosting your metabolism and losing fat is a slow process with no shortcuts. However, if you achieve that and become a master of it you will never have to worry about it, ever again. Most of the tips that I am about to offer you, will help you to improve every aspect of your life. It's like hitting 2000 birds with one stone so losing a bunch of weight will be the last thing you will worry about. Speaking of weight, let's clarify one main thing; forget the phrase "lose weight" and replace it with "lose fat" instead. Make sure you stick to the piece of advice I am about to provide you with, and I can guarantee to you that you will be rewarded in the long run.

To begin with, let's start with the understanding of what metabolism is. In a few words, it is the amount of energy that your body consumes. There are lots of factors that contribute to this, 3 of which you can't actually control. These are the following:

1. **Age:** Probably, you've already heard of this before; it's true that your metabolism gets slower as you age and that is because of muscle loss and hormonal changes.
2. **Gender:** typically, women tend to have slower metabolism due to their lower muscle to fat ratio, different hormones, and smaller size.
3. **Genetics:** this factor is completely unmeasurable since every person is different.

You want to hear my opinion? Well...just get over it. There is no reason to ruin your mood. Now, since time is money and I don't like to waste it, let's get down to business.

NUTRITION

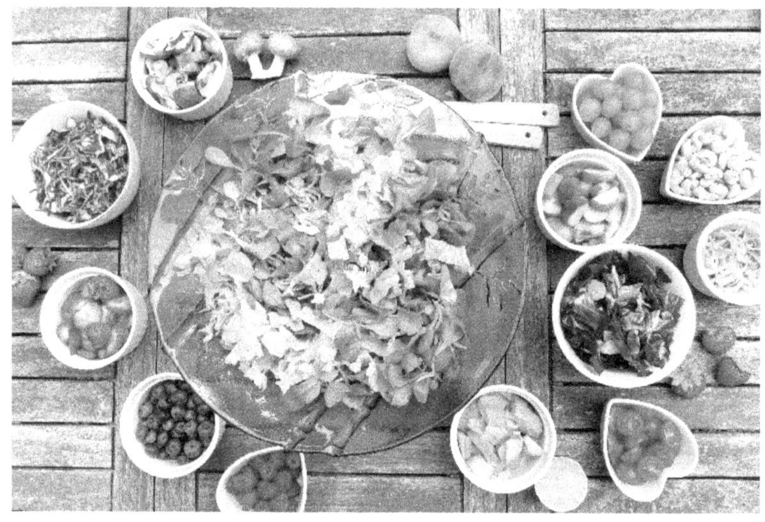

- **Carbohydrates:** AKA "carbs" are the main source of energy that your body uses. They are divided into two categories: simple and complex carbs; simple carbs are sugars and as you know they are not the healthiest thing you can consume. On the other hand, complex carbs are digested more slowly, offering you a steady amount of energy. In addition to that, they contain a lot of fiber which is not only essential for your health but also boosts your metabolism, as well.

Simple carbs: everything that contains sugar, are the ones you need to avoid.

Complex carbs: whole grains, vegetables, oats, and brown rice

- ☐ **Fats:** Fats are the most important part of your diet because they control your hormone levels and are essential for the proper function of your brain and your body organs. Just like carbs, fats are, also, divided into "good" ones and "bad" ones. Saturated fats and trans fats are the ones you should avoid at any cost as they are linked to some of the most serious diseases such as diabetes, heart disease, cardiovascular disease, and obesity.
  Monounsaturated and polyunsaturated are considered the "good" fats and they can be digested a lot easier by your system. As a result, they can help you to improve your metabolism.
  Saturated and trans fats: vegetable oils, processed food, and junk food, in general
  Monounsaturated and polyunsaturated fats: fish oil, omega 3 oil, olive oil, avocado, peanut butter, almonds, and cashews

- **Proteins:** you need to include an adequate amount of protein in every meal (ideally about 20-30 grams). There are 2 main reasons for this. The first one is that it makes you feel full, reduces your appetite and overall gives you a saturated feeling. The second one is that it has a higher thermic effect than carbs and fats, which means that your body needs more energy to break them down. In addition to that, make sure you include a variety of different protein sources in your diet so as to obtain all the essential amino acids.
The best protein sources: fish, egg whites, chicken, red meat, turkey, milk, cottage cheese, greek yogurt, lentils, and beans

- **Vitamins:** the following ones have a direct impact on your metabolism:
    - **B1:** It helps the body cells convert carbohydrates into energy and it can be found in pork, salmon, brown rice, mussels, and asparagus
    - **B2:** It helps metabolize glucose and it can be found in eggs, avocado, nuts, dairy products, and meat
    - **B6:** It helps metabolize protein and it can be found in milk, carrots, spinach, bananas, and tuna
    - **C:** It helps metabolize fat molecules and it can be found in kale, broccoli, lemons, oranges, and kiwi
    - **D:** It helps your body retain minerals and it can be found in sardines, mushrooms, liver oil, sun, and salmon
    - **K:** It helps produce prothrombin that improves blood clotting and bone metabolism and it can be found in swiss chard, chicken, green beans, parsley, and kale

- **Minerals** play an important role in boosting your metabolism:
    - **zinc:** It boosts your immune system, it helps protein and DNA synthesis and it improves skin and hair health. It can be found in meat, shellfish, whole grains seeds, and nuts.
    - **iron:** It helps your body carry oxygen to all of its cells and it can be found in spinach, legumes, red meat, quinoa, and tofu.
    - **calcium:** It increases your body's core temperature which as a result, it makes it burn more calories. It can be found in seeds, cheese, almonds, rhubarb, and figs.
    - **magnesium:** It helps in blood sugar regulation, muscle contraction building, and maintaining healthy teeth and bones. It can be found in dark chocolate, nuts, bananas, avocados, and tuna.

- **Capsaicin:** It is an active component, found in spicy foods that raises your metabolic rate. Metabolic rate affects the speed at which your body converts food into energy. Another way through which it boosts your metabolism is by increasing the temperature of your body and making it burn more calories. It, also, reduces insulin levels which is a hormone causing fat storage and muscle loss. Some foods that contain capsaicin are: jalapeño peppers, cayenne peppers, and red peppers.

- **Probiotics:** Probiotics contain enzymes and bacteria that increase levels of fat-regulating proteins and releasing appetite-regulating hormones which enables you to burn more fat. Foods that contain probiotics are the following: yogurt, sauerkraut, tempeh, kefir, kimchi, gouda, mozzarella, and buttermilk.

A general rule of thumb is to prefer unprocessed over-processed food since your body needs more energy to metabolize it and it has many beneficial results for your health, too.

Now, here is what you should avoid drinking:

- **Alcohol:** This is non-negotiable as it includes a lot of empty calories that contain zero nutrients micronutrients and vitamins. Moreover, it increases insulin levels that, as I said before, is a hormone you want to keep at a low level. Besides, it affects your digestion and nutrient intake. Not convinced yet? just search on google.

- **Artificial sweeteners:** Something that might haven't crossed your mind, is that diet sodas and drinks with 0 calories are actually very unhealthy, as well. That's because they contain artificial sweeteners that increase insulin levels. In addition to that, they are linked to metabolic syndrome which as its name implies, can't be very good.

Instead, prefer the following:

- **Water:** And especially the moment that you wake up to hydrate your body after all the hours of sleep you had. Cold water, actually, has the extra benefit to decrease your body's core temperature, which forces it to burn more calories. Try to drink between 2-4 liters per day.

- **Caffeine:** Adding a cup of coffee in the morning can increase the number of calories your body burns throughout the day. You can also get a similar effect to this with cacao and teas that, also, contain caffeine, such as black and green tea. Just don't over do it because it can lead to dehydration.

TRAINING

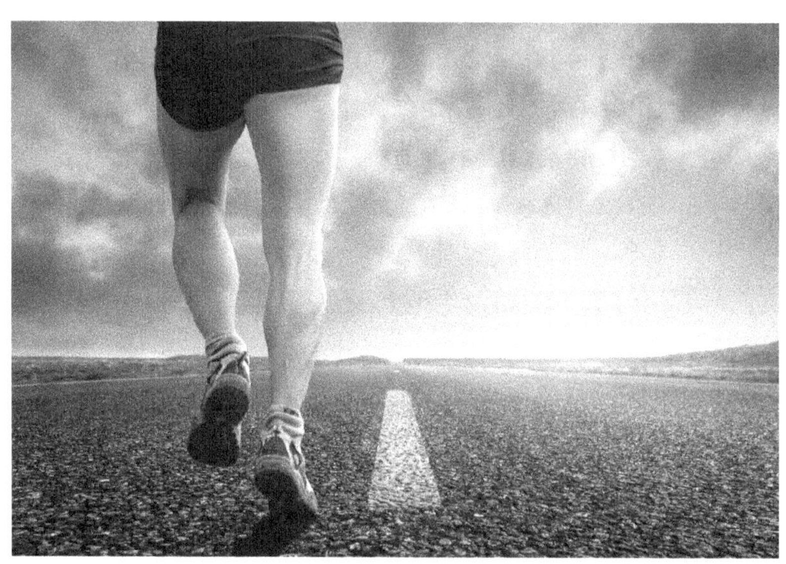

My favorite part and the most fun, in my opinion, because it has so many benefits.

- **Building muscle:** Having more muscle requires more energy to maintain it, using this extra muscle also requires more energy. You can think of it like a car; the bigger it is the more gas it needs to move. So how do you build muscle? By lifting heavy weight, of course! Doing it will not only increase your muscle but also your testosterone, which is a hormone that counters insulin. All this is an upward spiral. The hardest thing is to get in.

Best compound exercises: Deadlifts, Squats, Pull-ups, Barbell bench press, Military presses, and Dips.

Best isolation exercises for

- Chest: Dumbbell flyes, Crossover, DB pullover
- Back: Dumbbell row, Seated back extension, Cable straight-arm pulldown
- Legs: Hamstring curls, Leg extensions, Calf raises
- Triceps: Tricep pushdown, Cable overhead tricep extension, Barbell skullcrushers
- Biceps: Concentration curls, Barbell curls, Hammer curls
- Shoulders: Reverse flyes, Dumbbell lateral raise, Dumbbell front raise
- Abdominals: Russian twists, Vertical leg crunches, Reverse crunches

- **HITT:** It is an acronym for High-Intensity interval training. It's basically a high-intensity, low rest workout that targets your cardiovascular system and improves your athletic capacity. It, also, increases glucose metabolism which maximizes the number of calories you burn. Combine a lot of exercises in one set, add some resistance to them and keep your rest time between 30-45 seconds. Every individual is different, so feel free to adjust the program to your level. But keep in mind that the key here is to exhaust yourself and reach your limits.

- **Cardio:** But you have to learn to do it the right way. First, you have to calculate your max BPM. Max BPM stands for maximum beats per minute and it's basically your maximum heart rate. To calculate this, you subtract 220-(your age) for example if you are 20 years old it's 200.
The ideal rate for fat loss is between 60-80% of max BPM for the example above it's between 120-160 beats per minute. Keep your heart rate to those levels for at least 20 minutes to a maximum of one hour for the best possible results.

LIFESTYLE CHANGES

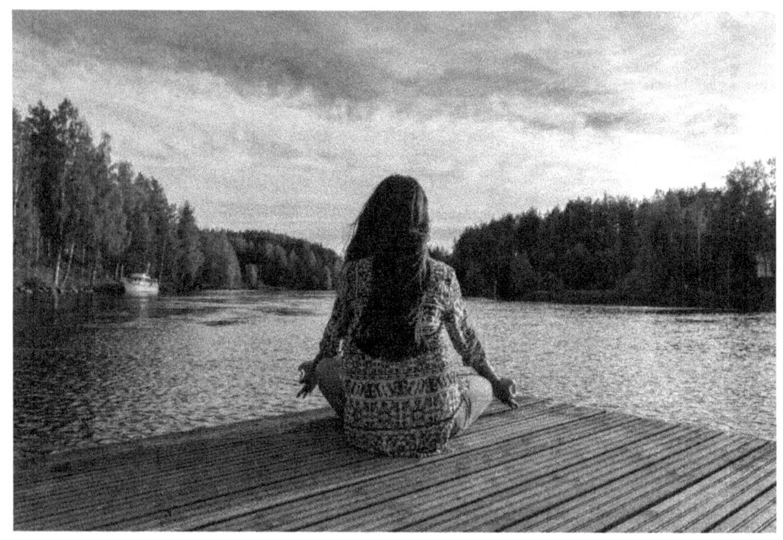

Lifestyle changes are going to be the easiest and the fastest way to see results. The key here is to start and make improvements as you go.

- **Meals:** Don't skip your meals, there is nothing you can do to make up for that. If you eat more on the next meal you are raising your insulin levels. On the other hand, if you don't eat the lost calories at all, you harm your metabolism by being in a caloric deposit. As I mentioned before, eating big meals raises your insulin levels so try avoiding it by splitting your food into smaller meals throughout the day.
Along with that, strive to eat your meals at the same time every day, as studies have found that this reduces cholesterol and insulin levels.

- **Cutting calories:** This one is very important! DO NOT cut calories or exhaust yourself through extreme diets. This mistake is so common and I see it all the time.

  Even though you might see some quick results, it is not sustainable for a long period of time and it will end up destroying your effort much more than it's going to benefit you. Just think about it: Is it worth losing 5 or 10 pounds at the cost of cutting what you eat in half? And also can you do this forever? Since once you start eating normally again, you are going to gain back all the weight. This strategy is simply deceiving from every point of view.

- **Daily activity:** Be as active as possible throughout your day. That includes the following cliches like skipping the elevator and taking the stairs, or going for a walk with your dog (if you have), or even going by foot instead of driving. In addition to that, you can burn a few more calories, by simply standing instead of sitting.

- **Stress management:** Lowering your stress levels is also a really good way not only to increase your metabolism but also to improve every aspect of your life. And, especially in modern times, that many people suffer from conditions based on this. I could write a different book just focused on that specific topic. Anyway, some good ways to reduce stress are the following: exercise, meditation, and my personal favorite, deep house music.

- **Smoking:** And for God's sake: DONT SMOKE! Do I really have to explain to you why?

- **Sleep:** The last piece of advice I want to give you is about sleep. Try sleeping for 7-8 daily, preferably at night, and avoid short naps. Increase the quality of your sleep and the calories you burn by lowering the temperature of the room. And start using blue light blockers on your screens a few hours before you go to bed so as to keep your melatonin in normal levels.
Ways to improve sleep quality even more: Sleep in a pitch-black room, wake up the same time every day, don't drink caffeine 8 hours before bedtime, wear earplugs.

CONCLUSION

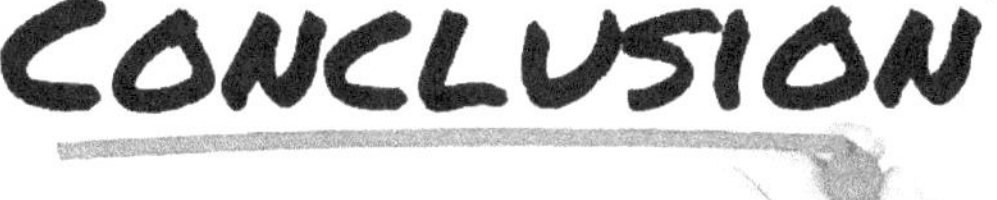

I know what you might be thinking; a lot of the above tips didn't come to you as a surprise and you probably, already, knew them. However, be honest with yourself: how many of them are you actually following, and, even if you do, how often? The purpose of this book is not to give a secret recipe that will make you lose 20 pounds in just one week. Instead, It is to get you on the right mindset; In other words, working for yourself is a lifelong process and this book aims to remind you of all the things that you should do for yourself and, hopefully, inspire you and motivate you to take action. Of course, some tips are way more effective than others. Are you ready to learn which one is the best? And the winner is... Cardio! And in particular with an empty stomach as soon as you wake up. All you have to do is to drink a lot of water as soon as you wake up and then go for cardio fasted. After you finish, proceed to your daily routine.

Thank You for purchasing and reading this book, I hope it was able to help you take control of your metabolism and archive all your fitness goals.

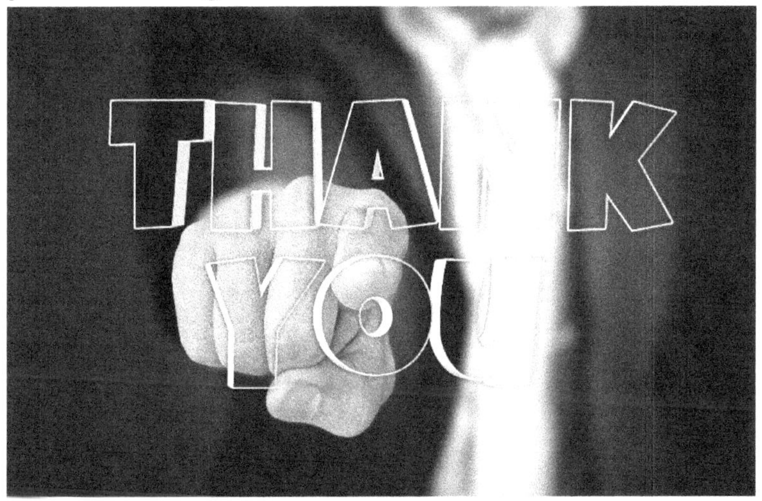

If you enjoyed the book, leave an honest review on Amazon. This will help motivate me to improve my content and provide higher quality products in the future.